The

Low

TESTOSTERONE

Fix

The complete cookbook to boost testosterone in men above 60

Dr. Ben Isaacson

Table Of Contents

Copyright

Disclaimer

Introduction

What is Testosterone?

Diet Basics For Boosting Testosterone

Testosterone Meal Plan And Recipes

Lifestyle changes for increasing testosterone

Supplements And Medications for Low Testosterone

Conclusion

Copyright

Disclaimer

The information in this book is not intended to be a substitute for professional medical advice, diagnosis, or treatment. Always seek the advice of your physician or other qualified healthcare providers with any questions you may have regarding a medical condition

Introduction

Testosterone is a hormone that is produced primarily in the testicles in men and the ovaries in women, although small amounts are also produced by the adrenal glands. It is responsible for the development of male sex organs and secondary male characteristics such as facial hair, a deeper voice, and a muscular build. In women, testosterone is produced in smaller amounts and plays a role in maintaining bone density, sex drive, and cognitive function.

Testosterone levels naturally decline with age in both men and women. In men, testosterone levels generally peak during adolescence and early adulthood and then gradually decline with age.

Testosterone is a male hormone that plays a key role in many of the body's functions, including muscle mass, bone density, and sexual function. As men, agmedicationterone levels naturally decrease. Low testosterone levels in men, also known as hypogonadism, can cause symptoms such as low sex drive, decreased bone density, fatigue, and decreased muscle mass.

This low testosterone cookbook is a collection of recipes that are designed to help men over the age of 60 who have low testosterone levels. These recipes include ingredients that are known to increase testosterone production or support overall testosterone health. Some examples of these ingredients include:

Zinc: This mineral is essential for testosterone production and can be found in foods like oysters, red meat, and beans.

Magnesium: Magnesium is another mineral that is important for testosterone production and can be found in foods like nuts, whole grains, and leafy green vegetables.

Healthy fats: Healthy fats, such as those found in avocados, olive oil, and nuts, are important for hormone production and overall health.

Protein: Adequate protein intake is important for maintaining muscle mass, which is important for testosterone health. Good sources of protein include meat, fish, eggs, and dairy products.

It's important to note that while this low testosterone cookbook can be a helpful resource, it is not a substitute for medical treatment. If you are concerned about your testosterone levels, it is important to speak with a healthcare professional.

What is Testosterone?

Testosterone is the hormone liable for the advancement of male sexual qualities. Hormones are chemical messengers that trigger essential changes in the body. Females likewise produce testosterone, normally in small amounts.

Testosterone is a kind of androgen created principally by the testicles in cells called the Leydig cells.
In men, testosterone is thought to manage various functions alongside sperm production. These include:

- sex drive
- bone mass
- fat circulation

- muscle size and strength
- red blood cell production

Without sufficient measures of testosterone, men become infertile. This is because testosterone helps the maturation of sperm.

Despite being a male sex hormone, testosterone likewise adds to sex drive, bone thickness, and muscle strength in ladies. Notwithstanding, an excess of testosterone can likewise make ladies experience male pattern hair sparseness (baldness) and infertility.

The brain and pituitary gland manage testosterone levels. When produced, the hormone travels through the blood to carry out its various significant functions.

Why is it important?

- It is responsible for the development of male sex organs and secondary sexual characteristics, such as facial hair and a deeper voice.

- It helps maintain muscle mass and strength.

- It plays a role in bone density and the maintenance of strong bones.

- It helps regulate the production of red blood cells.

- It plays a role in the production of sperm and the maintenance of fertility.

- It helps regulate mood and mental function.

- It helps regulate metabolism and body weight.

- It plays a role in the development of the prostate gland and the maintenance of prostate health.

- It helps regulate the immune system.

- It plays a role in sexual desire in both men and women.

- It helps regulate cholesterol levels in the body.

- It assists in blood pressure regulation.

- It plays a role in the development of lean body mass.

- It might help to reduce the risk of cardiovascular disease.

- It may help reduce the risk of type 2 diabetes.

- It may help improve memory and cognitive function.

- It may help reduce the risk of depression and anxiety.

- It may help improve sleep quality.

- It might help to improve cardiovascular health.

- It may help reduce the risk of osteoporosis

It's important to note that while testosterone has many important functions in the body, it is also possible to have too much or too little of it. Abnormal levels of testosterone can cause a variety of health problems and should be monitored and managed by a healthcare professional.

What are the symptoms of low testosterone in men over 60?

Several symptoms can indicate low testosterone in men. Some of the most common symptoms include:

- Low sex drive
- Erectile dysfunction
- Fatigue
- Decreased muscle mass and strength
- Increased body fat
- Mood changes, including depression and irritability
- Difficulty concentrating
- Poor sleep
- Decreased bone density
- Decreased sperm count
- Smaller testicles
- Breast enlargement
- Decreased body hair
- Hot flashes
- Lowered energy levels
- Decreased mental sharpness
- Difficulty building muscle
- Loss of the body or facial hair
- Decreased self-confidence
- Changes in cholesterol levels
- Difficulty remembering things
- Loss of height
- Mood swings
- Decreased sense of well-being
- Decreased ability to perform physical activities
- Lack of motivation
- Loss of interest in work or other activities
- Decreased enthusiasm for life
- Decreased ability to handle stress
- Decreased enjoyment of life
- Decreased ability to cope with stress
- Irritability
- Anxiety

- Depression
- Decreased sense of accomplishment
- Decreased sense of purpose in life
- Decreased sense of belonging
- Decreased sense of control over life
- Decreased sense of personal worth
- Decreased sense of achievement
- Difficulty maintaining relationships
- Social isolation
- Decreased participation in activities
- Decreased enjoyment of hobbies and other activities
- Decreased ability to take pleasure in life
- Decreased satisfaction with life
- Decreased sense of connection to others
- Decreased sense of community
- Decreased sense of security
- Decreased sense of safety

What are the causes of low testosterone in men above 60?

There are many potential causes of low testosterone in men above the age of 60. Some possible causes include:

Aging: Testosterone levels naturally decline with age.

Obesity: Being overweight or obese can lead to low testosterone levels.

Chronic illness: Chronic illnesses such as diabetes, HIV, and liver or kidney disease can cause low testosterone.

Alcohol consumption: Heavy alcohol consumption can lead to low testosterone levels.

Stress: Chronic stress can lead to decreased testosterone production.

Sleep deprivation: Not getting enough sleep can lower testosterone levels.

Medications: Some medications, such as steroids and opioids, can suppress testosterone production.

Hypogonadism: This is a condition in which the body does not produce enough testosterone. It can be caused by problems with the testicles, pituitary gland, or hypothalamus.

Klinefelter syndrome: This is a genetic disorder that affects male sexual development and can lead to low testosterone levels.

Undescended testicles: If a baby boy's testicles do not descend into the scrotum before birth, it can lead to low testosterone levels later in life.

Testicle injury or infection: Testicles produce testosterone, so any injury or infection that affects them can lead to low testosterone levels.

Hemochromatosis: This is a condition in which the body absorbs too much iron, which can damage the testicles and lead to low testosterone levels.

Inflammation: Chronic inflammation in the body can interfere with testosterone production.

Pituitary gland problems: The pituitary gland helps regulate testosterone production. If it is not functioning properly, testosterone levels may be low.

Poor nutrition: A lack of certain nutrients, such as zinc and vitamin D, can contribute to low testosterone levels.

Tumors: Tumors in the pituitary gland, testicles, or adrenal gland can lead to low testosterone levels.

Trauma: Physical trauma, such as a car accident or injury, can damage the testicles and lead to low testosterone levels.

This is not a complete list, but rather a selection of some of the more common causes of low testosterone in men over 60. If you are experiencing low testosterone, it is important to speak with a healthcare provider to determine the cause and receive proper treatment.

What are the benefits of increased testosterone levels in men above 60?

Testosterone is a hormone that is produced by the testicles in men and is responsible for the development of male characteristics, such as facial hair and a deep voice. It also plays a role in maintaining muscle mass and bone density, as well as sex drive. As men get older, their testosterone levels naturally dwindle. Some potential benefits of increasing testosterone levels in men over 60 may include:

Improved muscle mass and strength: Testosterone plays a role in building and maintaining muscle mass, so increasing testosterone levels may help older men maintain or even increase their muscle mass and strength.

Increased bone density: Testosterone plays a role in maintaining bone density, so increasing testosterone levels may help older men maintain or even increase their bone density, which can help prevent osteoporosis.

Improved sexual function: Testosterone is important for maintaining sex drive, so increasing testosterone levels may help improve sexual function in older men.

Improved mood: Low testosterone levels have been linked to a decrease in mood and an increase in depression in older men, so increasing testosterone levels may help improve mood.

Improved cognition: Some studies have suggested that increasing testosterone levels may help improve cognitive function in older men.

Others are:

- Increased red blood cell production
- Improved cardiovascular health
- Increased hair growth
- Improved sleep
- Increased self-esteem and confidence
- Improved prostate health
- Increased insulin sensitivity
- Improved blood sugar control
- Improved heart health
- Improved skin health
- Increased energy levels
- Improved memory
- Improved immune function
- Enhanced athletic performance
- Improved quality of life

It's important to note that the benefits of increasing testosterone levels may vary from person to person and that more research is needed to fully understand the potential risks and benefits of testosterone replacement therapy. If you are considering testosterone replacement therapy, it's important to talk to your doctor to determine if it is right for you.

Diet Basics For Boosting Testosterone

When you adopt and maintain a healthy diet, it benefits your testosterone levels in two primary ways:

- Enhances weight loss and a healthy weight
- Decreases the chance of increased blood sugar

Males who are obese are much more likely to have low levels of testosterone. Excess fat in the abdomen is likely a major culprit. Having more of this type of fat is considered to lead to a higher production of the enzyme known as aromatase, which converts testosterone into estradiol — lowering a man's free testosterone levels. As a result of this, shedding weight may enhance testosterone levels, and a healthy diet can assist you to achieve that.

A balanced diet includes plenty of vegetables and fruits, whole-grain carbohydrates, moderate amounts of healthy fats, and lean protein, such as chicken and fish.

The key to a balanced diet when trying to increase your testosterone levels is to avoid refined, simple carbohydrates, like the ones found in chips and other junk food. These simple carbohydrates can lead to spikes in your blood sugar and have been shown to reduce free testosterone levels.

Macronutrients: Proteins, Carbohydrates, and Fats

There is no direct role of protein, carbohydrates, or fats in boosting testosterone levels. Testosterone is a hormone produced by the body, and its production is complex and regulated by various factors, including genetics, age, and overall health. However, a healthy and balanced diet can help to support overall hormone health, including testosterone production.

Proteins: Revealed to give satiety following a meal, the amino acids in protein likewise support fat-consuming and muscle recuperation post-exercise. You'll need a decent part of your eating routine - around 25% to 35% - to come from protein-based sources like chicken, hamburger, yogurt, and pumpkin seeds.

Carbohydrates: Diets that are lower in entire carbohydrates and just focus on complex sources, for example, dark leafy green vegetables and entire grains have been revealed to help testosterone production. The exemption for this would be if you are constantly involved in an exercise program. Studies show that post-exercise carbohydrate utilization following extreme exercise can support free testosterone levels and put cortisol levels under control.

On the off chance that you are not very active, you might need to consider a low-carb diet; one where carbs just make up 10% to 25% of the all-out caloric admission. Atkins and the ketogenic diet are incredible models.

If you are a very active person, you might need to eat a higher level of complex carbohydrate sources, for example, 30% to 45%.

Fats: Regardless of the terrible publicity that dietary fats once got, countless studies have shown the significant role of healthy fatty acids in keeping a healthy weight, yet more importantly, healthy testosterone levels. Studies show that eating an adequate number of sound fats every day is critical to supporting elevated degrees of testosterone.

How much fat you eat each day relies upon which kind of diet you pick. A lower-carb diet will normally have more fat substances. For instance, if you're following a ketogenic diet, 60% to 80% of your all-out caloric intake will come from fat. If you are following a moderate-carb diet, 30% to 40% of your calories might come from fat.

Regardless of which diet you pick, there are a few food sources that can either positively or negatively affect your testosterone levels.

Micronutrients: Vitamins, Minerals, and Antioxidants.

Micronutrients are essential nutrients that the body needs in small amounts to function properly. These include vitamins and minerals such as zinc, magnesium, and vitamin D. These micronutrients play a role in many bodily processes, including the production of testosterone.

Zinc is a mineral that is essential for the production of testosterone. It is also involved in the proper functioning of the immune system and wound healing. Some good sources of zinc include oysters, beef, pumpkin seeds, and chickpeas.

Boron as a mineral has been shown to increase testosterone levels and improve other markers of hormonal health in men

Magnesium is another mineral that is important for testosterone production. It is also involved in protein synthesis and energy production. Some good sources of magnesium include nuts, leafy green vegetables, and whole grains.

Vitamin K2 is a type of vitamin K that is found in certain animal-derived foods and fermented foods. It is important for the proper functioning of the body's blood clotting system and for maintaining healthy bones.
Good sources of vitamin K2 include:

Cheese, particularly hard cheeses such as Gouda, Brie, and Edam
Egg yolks, particularly from chickens that have been fed a diet rich in vitamin K2
Meat, particularly organ meats such as liver and kidney
Fermented foods: such as natto (a type of fermented soybean), sauerkraut, and pickles

Vitamin D is a hormone that is produced by the body when the skin is exposed to sunlight. It is important for bone health and may also play a role in testosterone production. Some good sources of vitamin D include fatty fish, mushrooms, and fortified foods like milk and cereal.

Anti-oxidants

There is some evidence that certain antioxidants may play a role in regulating testosterone levels and improving fertility in men. For example, vitamin C, a potent antioxidant, has been shown to increase testosterone levels in animals. Additionally, a study of men with fertility issues found that taking an antioxidant supplement containing vitamin C, vitamin E, and selenium improved sperm motility and decreased oxidative stress. However, it's important to note that more research is needed to fully understand the relationship between antioxidants and testosterone. It's also worth noting that while antioxidants may have some beneficial effects on testosterone levels and fertility, they are not a substitute for proper medical treatment and should not be used as such. If you have concerns about your testosterone levels or fertility, it's important to speak with a healthcare professional.

It is important to get enough of these micronutrients in your diet to support optimal testosterone production and overall health. However, it is also important to note that testosterone levels can be affected by many other factors, such as age, weight, and underlying health conditions. If you are concerned about your testosterone levels, it is important to speak with a healthcare professional for personalized advice.

Hydration and Testosterone

Testosterone is a hormone produced by the testicles in males and, to a lesser extent, the ovaries in females. It plays a key role in the development of male sexual characteristics, such as facial and pubic hair, deepened voice, and increased muscle mass. It also helps to maintain bone density and sperm production.

Proper hydration is important for overall health and can also play a role in maintaining healthy testosterone levels. Dehydration can cause a decrease in testosterone levels, which can lead to decreased libido, fertility, and muscle mass. In severe cases, dehydration can also cause more serious health problems.

On the other hand, proper hydration may help to support healthy testosterone production and function. Adequate hydration can help to maintain healthy blood volume and ensure that the body has sufficient fluids to support the physiological processes that produce testosterone. To stay hydrated, you must drink enough fluids, especially water.

Importance of staying hydrated

Maintains healthy blood volume: Adequate hydration is important for maintaining healthy blood volume, which is important for maintaining healthy testosterone levels.

Supports testosterone production: Proper hydration can help to support the physiological processes that produce testosterone.

Helps to maintain muscle mass: Testosterone plays a role in maintaining muscle mass, and proper hydration can help to support this process.

Maintains bone density: Testosterone helps to maintain bone density, and proper hydration can help to support this process.

Supports sperm production: Testosterone is important for maintaining sperm production, and proper hydration can help to support this process.

Maintains libido: Testosterone is important for maintaining libido, and proper hydration can help to support healthy testosterone levels and libido.

Maintains fertility: Testosterone is important for fertility, and proper hydration can help to support healthy testosterone levels and fertility.

Helps to prevent dehydration: Dehydration can cause a decrease in testosterone levels, so proper hydration can help to prevent this from occurring.

Supports overall health: Adequate hydration is important for overall health, and maintaining healthy testosterone levels is just one aspect of this.

Importance of staying hydrated to testosterone

- Staying hydrated helps to regulate body temperature.
- Dehydration can lead to fatigue, which can decrease testosterone levels.
- Adequate hydration is necessary for proper blood flow, which is important for hormone transport and delivery.
- Dehydration can cause an increase in the hormone cortisol, which can negatively affect testosterone levels.
- Hydration is necessary for proper kidney function, which is important for maintaining healthy testosterone levels.
- Adequate hydration can help to maintain healthy digestion and absorption of nutrients, which are necessary for healthy testosterone production.
- Dehydration can cause muscle cramps, which can disrupt workouts and affect testosterone production.
- Staying hydrated can help to maintain healthy blood pressure, which is important for overall health and testosterone production.
- Hydration is necessary for proper brain function, which can affect mood and energy levels, which in turn can affect testosterone levels.
- Adequate hydration can help to maintain healthy skin, which can affect body image and self-esteem, which are important for healthy testosterone levels.
- Hydration is necessary for proper immune function, which is important for maintaining overall health and healthy testosterone production.
- Dehydration can cause headaches, which can affect mood and energy levels, which can in turn affect testosterone levels.
- Staying hydrated can help to prevent constipation, which can affect hormone balance and testosterone production.

- Adequate hydration is necessary for the proper functioning of all organs and systems in the body, which is important for maintaining healthy testosterone levels.
- Dehydration can cause dry mouth and bad breath, which can affect social interactions and self-esteem, which can affect testosterone levels.
- Hydration is necessary for proper joint function, which is important for maintaining an active lifestyle and healthy testosterone production.
- Staying hydrated can help to maintain a healthy body weight, which is important for healthy testosterone levels.
- Adequate hydration can help to prevent urinary tract infections, which can affect overall health and testosterone production.
- Hydration is necessary for proper blood oxygenation, which is important for overall health and testosterone production.
- Staying hydrated can help to maintain healthy energy levels, which can affect physical activity and mood, which are vital for maintaining healthy testosterone levels.

Food varieties Supporting Testosterone Levels

Here are some of the best testosterone-supporting food sources that you can start adding to your eating routine:

- Entire eggs (with yolk)
- Pumpkin seeds
- Dark leafy greens and cruciferous vegetables (e.g., broccoli, kale, spinach)
- Fenugreek
- Grass-fed beef and lamb
- Maca
- Clam
- Ginger
- Ginseng

- Fish
- Crude honey
- Maca on a white foundation

Food varieties Bringing down Testosterone Levels

The following are a bunch of the most terrible food sources for testosterone levels:

- Soy and soy-based items (e.g., tofu)
- Flaxseed
- Liquor (e.g., high-calorie beers) and excessive drinking
- Simple, processed carbohydrates (e.g., sugar-based unhealthy foods)
- Trans-fat-based items (e.g., French fries from a drive-through joint or fast-food restaurant)
- Mint and spearmint
- Licorice
- Vegetable and canola oil
- Any food with an elevated degree of pesticides

Testosterone Meal Plan And Recipes

The following testosterone-supporting meal plan depends on one day and it incorporates some plant-based choices that are high in protein, fat, or both.

Breakfast:

2 entire eggs
½ cup of egg whites
3 portions of bacon
Greens smoothie with broccoli, kale, spinach, and maca

Early in the day Bite:
¾ cup of curds
½ cup of pumpkin seeds

Lunch:

5 ounces of chicken thighs, barbecued
1 cup of vegetable assortment (center around dull mixed greens)
2 tablespoons of olive oil (for vegetables)

Mid-Evening Bite:

2 scoops of whey protein disengage
1 tablespoon of chia (in the shake)
1 tablespoon of maca (in the shake)

Supper:

3 ounces of grass-took care of hamburger
1 cup of broccoli
1 tablespoon of grass-took care of margarine (for broccoli)

Testosterone Supporting Recipes

Not positive about the kitchen? That is completely fine! The
following are a couple of testosterone-supporting recipes that are
not difficult to make, extraordinary for your waistline, and are
successful in helping your t-levels.

Plant Flapjacks
Fixings:

1 ready banana
1 scoop of veggie-lover protein
1/2 cup oats

1/2 cup almond or coconut milk
1/4 cup almond flour to thicken
1 teaspoon normal vanilla (discretionary)

Directions:

Place everything into a blender
Mix on mode for 30 seconds
Oil a dish
Empty hitter into the dish
Cook on medium-high intensity for one to two minutes on each side

Ketogenic Meatballs
Fixings:

1/2 lb. ground hamburger
1/2 lb. ground sheep
1 ounce of garlic, minced
½ cup Parmesan
2 tbsp. Parsley
1 tbsp. onion salt
1 enormous egg, beaten
1 tsp. ocean salt
1/2 tsp. dark pepper
2 tbsp. extra-virgin olive oil

Guidelines:

Join the egg, preparation, and cheddar with the meat
Blend the meat in with your hands
Structure into 10 to 18 meatballs, contingent upon the inclination
Cook the meatballs in a skillet over medium-high intensity for around 10 minutes

Protein Avocado Frozen yogurt
Fixings:

1 avocado, no skin or seed
1 scoop of whey protein (your number one flavor)
1 cup of ice
1 cup of almond, coconut, or normal milk

Directions:

Place every one of the fixings into a blender
Mix on high for around 30 seconds
Place in the freezer for a couple of hours
Enjoy

Lifestyle changes for increasing testosterone

Lifestyle changes for increasing testosterone refer to modifications to your daily habits and routines that may help boost testosterone levels. Testosterone is a hormone that plays a key role in the development and maintenance of male sexual characteristics, as well as muscle mass, bone density, and red blood cell production. Several lifestyle changes may help increase testosterone levels, such as exercising regularly, eating a healthy diet, getting enough sleep, managing stress, limiting alcohol intake, and avoiding environmental toxins. It's important to note that these lifestyle changes may help increase testosterone levels, but they are not a substitute for medical treatment if you have a deficiency or other medical condition. If you are concerned about your testosterone levels, it is best to speak with a healthcare provider.

Alcohol and Testosterone

There is evidence that alcohol consumption can reduce testosterone levels in men. Chronic heavy alcohol use has been linked to decreased testosterone production and decreased testicle size. Additionally, alcohol use can impair the release of testosterone from the testes, leading to decreased testosterone levels in the body. However, it is worth noting that the effects of alcohol on testosterone can vary depending on the individual and the amount of alcohol consumed. Some research suggests that moderate alcohol consumption may not significantly impact testosterone levels, but more research is needed to confirm this. It is generally recommended to consume alcohol in moderation, if at all, as excessive alcohol use can have many negative health effects.

Here are the potential effects of alcohol on testosterone:

Decreased testosterone production: Chronic heavy alcohol use has been linked to decreased testosterone production in the testes.

Decreased testicle size: Alcohol consumption has been shown to cause testicle shrinkage in animal studies.

Impaired release of testosterone from the testes: Alcohol use can disrupt the normal release of testosterone from the testes, leading to decreased testosterone levels in the body.

Decreased testosterone levels: Chronic heavy alcohol use has been linked to decreased testosterone levels in the body.

Increased estrogen levels: Alcohol consumption may increase estrogen levels in men, which can further decrease testosterone levels.

Decreased libido: Testosterone plays a role in libido, and decreased testosterone levels may result in a lower sex drive.

Erectile dysfunction: Testosterone is important for maintaining erectile function, and low testosterone levels can lead to erectile dysfunction.

Decreased muscle mass: Testosterone plays a role in muscle mass, and low testosterone levels may result in decreased muscle mass.

Increased body fat: Testosterone helps regulate body fat, and low testosterone levels may lead to increased body fat.

Decreased bone density: Testosterone is important for maintaining bone density, and low testosterone levels may result in decreased bone density and an increased risk of osteoporosis.

Exercise and Testosterone

Exercise has been shown to have a positive effect on testosterone levels in the body. Regular physical activity can increase testosterone production, particularly in response to weight training and high-intensity interval training.

Weight training is particularly effective at increasing testosterone levels. This may be because weight training increases the production of lactic acid, which has been shown to stimulate testosterone production.

High-intensity interval training (HIIT) has also been shown to be effective at increasing testosterone levels. This type of exercise involves short bursts of intense exercise followed by periods of rest. The short bursts of intense exercise help to increase testosterone production, while the periods of rest allow the body to recover and rebuild.

Overall, regular exercise can have several positive effects on testosterone levels and sexual function in men. It is important to speak with a healthcare provider before starting any exercise program, particularly if you have a medical condition or are taking any medications.

There are many benefits of exercise on testosterone levels, including:

Increased testosterone production: Exercise can increase testosterone production in the body, particularly in response to weight training and high-intensity interval training.

Improved sexual function: Testosterone plays a key role in sexual function, and research suggests that regular exercise can improve sexual function in men with low testosterone levels.

Enhanced muscle mass and strength: Testosterone plays a role in muscle growth and strength, and regular exercise can help to increase muscle mass and strength.

Improved body composition: Exercise can help to improve body composition by increasing muscle mass and reducing fat mass, which can have a positive effect on testosterone levels.

Increased energy levels: Testosterone can help to increase energy levels, and regular exercise can help to boost energy levels by improving overall fitness and stamina.

Improved mood: Testosterone has been linked to improved mood and a reduction in feelings of stress and anxiety. Exercise has also been shown to improve mood and reduce feelings of stress and anxiety.

Improved sleep: Testosterone is involved in the regulation of sleep, and regular exercise has been shown to improve sleep quality.

Improved cardiovascular health: Testosterone has a protective effect on the cardiovascular system, and regular exercise can help to improve cardiovascular health.

Improved cognitive function: Testosterone has been linked to improved cognitive function, and regular exercise has been shown to improve cognitive function in older adults.

Improved bone density: Testosterone plays a role in bone density, and regular exercise has been shown to improve bone density and reduce the risk of osteoporosis.

Sleep and Testosterone

There is a relationship between sleep and testosterone levels in the body. Testosterone is a hormone that plays a role in male development and is produced primarily in the testicles. It is also present, although to a lesser extent, in women. Testosterone levels in the body naturally fluctuate throughout the day and are generally highest in the morning and lowest at night.

Research has shown that men who get less sleep or have poor-quality sleep tend to have lower testosterone levels. One study found that men who slept for only 4 hours per night had testosterone levels that were 15% lower than men who slept for 8 hours per night. Another study found that men who experienced disrupted sleep due to sleep apnea had lower testosterone levels than men who slept uninterrupted.

In addition to its effects on testosterone, sleep is important for overall health and well-being. Getting enough quality sleep can help improve mood, memory, and physical performance. If you are having trouble sleeping, it is a good idea to speak with a healthcare provider to determine the cause and explore potential solutions.

Benefits of Sleep on Testosterone

There are several benefits of sleep on testosterone:

Sleep helps to regulate testosterone production. Testosterone levels are typically highest in the morning and lowest at night, and sleep is an important factor in this natural hormonal pattern.

Lack of sleep can lead to decreased testosterone levels. Men who don't get enough sleep may have lower testosterone levels than those who get enough sleep.

Sleep deprivation has been linked to lower libido. Testosterone is important for libido in both men and women, and men who don't get enough sleep may have a lower sex drive as a result.

Sleep may help improve muscle mass and strength. Testosterone plays a role in muscle growth and maintenance, and men who get enough sleep may have higher testosterone levels and therefore better muscle mass and strength.

Sleep may help improve athletic performance. Testosterone is important for physical performance, and men who get enough sleep may have higher testosterone levels and therefore better athletic performance.

Sleep may help improve mood. Testosterone is important for mood regulation in men, and men who don't get enough sleep may be more prone to mood problems such as irritability and depression.

Sleep may help improve cognitive function. Testosterone is important for brain function, and men who get enough sleep may have better memory, concentration, and problem-solving skills.

Sleep may help reduce the risk of obesity. Testosterone helps regulate body weight, and men who don't get enough sleep may be more likely to gain weight and become obese.

Sleep may help reduce the risk of heart disease. Testosterone helps regulate cholesterol levels, and men who don't get enough sleep may be more likely to develop heart disease.

Sleep may help reduce the risk of other health problems. Testosterone is important for overall health, and men who don't get enough sleep may be more likely to develop a range of other health problems.

Stress and Testosterone

Stress can affect testosterone levels in men. When a person is stressed, the body produces stress hormones such as cortisol. High levels of cortisol can decrease testosterone production. In addition, chronic stress can lead to unhealthy habits such as overeating, lack of exercise, and inadequate sleep, which can also contribute to low testosterone levels.

Effects of Stress on Testosterone

Stress can have several negative effects on testosterone levels in both men and women. Here are the potential effects of stress on testosterone:

Reduced testosterone production: Stress can suppress the production of testosterone in the body, leading to lower levels of the hormone.

Decreased sex drive: Testosterone plays a key role in libido, and stress can lower testosterone levels, which can lead to a decreased sex drive.

Erectile dysfunction: Testosterone is important for maintaining healthy erectile function, and stress can contribute to erectile dysfunction by lowering testosterone levels.

Decrease in muscle mass: Testosterone is essential for building and maintaining muscle mass, and low testosterone levels can lead to a decrease in muscle mass.

Increased body fat: Stress can lead to an increase in the production of the hormone cortisol, which can lead to an increase in body fat.

Decreased bone density: Testosterone plays a role in maintaining healthy bone density, and low testosterone levels can lead to decreased bone density and an increased risk of osteoporosis.

Decreased cognitive function: Testosterone is important for brain function, and low testosterone levels have been linked to decreased cognitive function and memory.

Depression: Low testosterone levels have been linked to an increased risk of depression.

Fatigue: Testosterone helps to regulate energy levels, and low testosterone levels can lead to fatigue and a lack of energy.

Irritability and mood changes: Testosterone plays a role in mood regulation, and low testosterone levels have been linked to irritability and mood changes.

Supplements And Medications for Low Testosterone

Supplements for low testosterone are products that are taken orally and are designed to help increase testosterone levels in the body. These supplements can be found over the counter and are not regulated by the Food and Drug Administration (FDA). Some examples of supplements that are claimed to increase testosterone levels include herbs, such as Tribulus Terrestris and fenugreek, as well as minerals, such as zinc and magnesium.

Medications for low testosterone, on the other hand, are prescription drugs that are designed to help increase testosterone levels in the body. These medications are regulated by the FDA and are generally considered to be more effective at increasing testosterone levels than supplements. Examples of medications that may be used to treat low testosterone include testosterone replacement therapy (TRT), clomiphene, human chorionic gonadotropin (HCG), and anastrozole.

Several supplements and medications can help to increase testosterone levels in men who have a deficiency. These include:

Testosterone replacement therapy (TRT): This involves taking testosterone in the form of injections, patches, gels, or pellets. TRT can be effective at increasing testosterone levels, but it can also have side effects, such as acne and changes in blood pressure.

Clomiphene: This medication can be taken by mouth and may help to increase testosterone levels in men with hypogonadism (low testosterone production).

Human chorionic gonadotropin (HCG): HCG is a hormone that can be taken by injection and may help to stimulate the production of testosterone in men with hypogonadism.

Anastrozole: This medication is used to treat breast cancer in women, but it may also be effective at reducing estrogen levels in men, which can help to increase testosterone levels.

It's important to speak with a healthcare provider before taking any supplements or medications for low testosterone. They can help to determine the cause of your low testosterone levels and recommend the most appropriate treatment.

Natural supplements for testosterone

Several natural supplements may help boost testosterone levels. However, it's important to note that these supplements are not a substitute for proper medical treatment and you should consult a healthcare professional before taking any supplements. Here are a few natural supplements that have been suggested to help increase testosterone levels:

Zinc: Zinc is an essential mineral that is found in a variety of foods, including oysters, beef, and beans. Some studies have suggested that zinc supplements may help to increase testosterone levels in men.

Vitamin D: Vitamin D is a fat-soluble vitamin that is important for the proper function of the immune system and the absorption of calcium. Some research suggests that low levels of vitamin D may be linked to low testosterone levels.

Deer antler velvet: Deer antler velvet is the soft, newly grown antler of male deer. It is believed to contain compounds that may help to increase testosterone levels.

Fenugreek: Fenugreek is a plant that is native to the Mediterranean region. It has been used for centuries as a natural remedy for a variety of conditions. Some studies have suggested that fenugreek supplements may help to increase testosterone levels.

Ashwagandha: Ashwagandha is an herb that has been used in Ayurvedic medicine for centuries. It is believed to help reduce stress and improve testosterone levels.

Tribulus Terrestris: Tribulus Terrestris is a plant that has been used in traditional medicine to treat a variety of conditions. Some studies have suggested that it may help to increase testosterone levels, although more research is needed to confirm this.

Tongkat Ali: Tongkat Ali is a plant that is native to Southeast Asia and has been traditionally used to enhance male fertility and libido. Some studies have suggested that it may help to increase testosterone levels.

D-aspartic acid: D-aspartic acid is an amino acid that is involved in the production of hormones such as testosterone. Some research suggests that D-aspartic acid supplements may help to increase testosterone levels, although more research is needed to confirm this.

Maca root: Maca root is a plant native to the Andes region of South America. It has been traditionally used to enhance fertility and libido. Some studies have suggested that maca root may help to increase testosterone levels.

Boron: Boron is a trace mineral that is found in a variety of foods, including nuts, beans, and fruits. Some research suggests that boron supplements may help to increase testosterone levels, although more research is needed to confirm this.

Panax ginseng: Panax ginseng is a plant that has been traditionally used in Asian medicine to enhance overall health and well-being. Some studies have suggested that it may help to increase testosterone levels, although more research is needed to confirm this.

Mucuna pruriens: Mucuna pruriens is a plant that has been traditionally used in Ayurvedic medicine to enhance fertility and libido. Some research suggests that it may help to increase testosterone levels.

Epimedium: Epimedium, also known as horny goat weed, is a plant that has been traditionally used to enhance libido and treat erectile dysfunction. Some studies have suggested that it may help to increase testosterone levels.

Chrysin: Chrysin is a flavonoid that is found in a variety of plants, including passionflower and chamomile. Some research suggests that chrysin supplements may help to increase testosterone levels, although more research is needed to confirm this.

Eurycoma longifolia: Eurycoma longifolia, also known as Tongkat Ali, is a plant that has been traditionally used to enhance male fertility and libido. Some studies have suggested that it may help to increase testosterone levels.

Ginger: Ginger is a common spice that has been traditionally used to treat a variety of conditions. Some research suggests that ginger may help to increase testosterone levels, although more research is needed to confirm this.

Rhodiola Rosea: Rhodiola Rosea is a plant that has been traditionally used to enhance physical and mental performance. Some research suggests that it may help to increase testosterone levels, although more research is needed to confirm this.

Yohimbe: Yohimbe is a plant that has been traditionally used to treat erectile dysfunction. Some studies have suggested that it may help to increase testosterone levels, although more research is needed to confirm this.

Korean red ginseng: Korean red ginseng is a type of ginseng that has been traditionally used in Asian medicine to enhance overall health and well-being. Some studies have suggested that it may help to increase testosterone levels, although more research is needed to confirm this.

Saw palmetto: Saw palmetto is a plant that has been traditionally used to treat symptoms of an enlarged prostate. Some research suggests that it may help to increase testosterone levels, although more research is needed to confirm this.

Nettle root: Nettle root is a plant that has been traditionally used to treat symptoms of an enlarged prostate. Some research suggests that it may help to increase testosterone levels, although more research is needed to confirm this.

Muira puama: Muira puama is a plant that has been traditionally used to enhance libido and treat erectile dysfunction. Some studies have suggested that it may help to increase testosterone levels.

Ginkgo biloba: Ginkgo biloba is a plant that has been traditionally used to enhance mental function and improve circulation. Some research suggests that it may help to increase testosterone levels, although more research is needed to confirm this.

L-arginine: L-arginine is an amino acid that is involved in the production of nitric oxide, which helps to relax blood vessels and improve circulation. Some research suggests that L-arginine supplements may help to increase testosterone levels, although more research is needed to confirm this.

Pycnogenol: Pycnogenol is a plant extract that is derived from the bark of the maritime pine tree. Some research suggests that it may help to increase testosterone levels, although more research is needed to confirm this.

Pine pollen: Pine pollen is a type of pollen that is collected from pine trees. Some research suggests that it may help to increase testosterone levels, although more research is needed to confirm this.

Cordyceps: Cordyceps is a type of mushroom that has been traditionally used in Chinese medicine to enhance overall health and well-being. Some research suggests that it may help to increase testosterone levels, although more research is needed to confirm this.

Shilajit: Shilajit is a resin-like substance that is found in the mountains of Asia. It has been traditionally used in Ayurvedic medicine to enhance overall well-being.

It's important to note that the effectiveness of these supplements may vary and more research is needed to fully understand their potential benefits and risks. As with any supplement, it's always a good idea to talk to a healthcare professional before starting a new supplement regimen.

Prescription medication for low testosterone

Prescription medications for low testosterone, also known as testosterone replacement therapy, are designed to help people whose bodies are not producing enough testosterone. Some common prescription medications for low testosterone include:

- Testosterone gels, such as AndroGel and Testim, are applied to the skin daily
- Testosterone patches, such as Androderm, are applied to the skin daily
- Testosterone injections, which are typically given in the muscle every two to four weeks
- Testosterone pellets, which are small pellets that are inserted under the skin every three to six months
- Testosterone nasal gels, such as Natesto, are applied to the inside of the nostrils daily

It's important to note that testosterone replacement therapy is only recommended for men who have low testosterone levels due to a medical condition, such as hypogonadism, and not for men who have low testosterone due to aging. Testosterone replacement therapy can have serious side effects and is not appropriate for everyone. It's important to discuss the risks and benefits with a healthcare provider before starting testosterone replacement therapy.

Pros of low testosterone supplements

Low testosterone, or low T, is a condition in which a man's body produces lower-than-normal levels of testosterone, the primary male sex hormone. Some potential benefits of using supplements or other treatments to increase testosterone levels include:

Improved libido: Low T can cause a decrease in sexual desire, and testosterone replacement therapy may help increase libido.

Improved muscle mass and strength: Testosterone plays a role in muscle mass and strength, and low T may cause a decline in muscle mass. Testosterone replacement therapy may help increase muscle mass and strength.

Improved bone density: Testosterone helps maintain bone density, and low T may increase the risk of osteoporosis. Testosterone replacement therapy may help improve bone density.

Improved mood: Low T can cause mood changes, such as increased irritability and depression. Testosterone replacement therapy may help improve mood.

Improved cognitive function: Some research suggests that testosterone may have a positive effect on cognitive function, including memory and processing speed.

It's important to note that testosterone supplements are not suitable for everyone, and it is important to speak with a healthcare provider before starting any treatment for low T.

Cons of low testosterone supplements

There are several potential drawbacks to using testosterone supplements. Here are a few:

Side effects: Testosterone supplements can cause a range of side effects, including acne, breast swelling, and increased aggression.

Health risks: Long-term use of testosterone supplements may increase the risk of heart attack, stroke, and prostate cancer.

Interactions with other medications: Testosterone supplements can interact with certain medications, such as blood thinners, and may cause unintended side effects.

Dependence: Some people may become dependent on testosterone supplements and may experience withdrawal symptoms when they stop using them.

Cost: Testosterone supplements can be expensive and may not be covered by insurance.

It's important to discuss the potential risks and benefits of testosterone supplements with a healthcare provider before starting treatment.

Pros of Testosterone Medications

- Improving sex drive and libido
- Increasing muscle mass and strength
- Improving bone density
- Reducing body fat
- Improving mood and well-being
- Improving the quality of life
- Increasing energy levels
- Enhancing cognitive function
- Improving sleep quality

- Improving cardiovascular health

Cons of Testosterone Medications

Testosterone replacement therapy (TRT) is a treatment for men with low testosterone levels. It is available in several forms, including gels, injections, and patches. While TRT can be effective in improving symptoms of low testosterone, it can also have some downsides. Here are ten potential cons of testosterone medications:

Risk of blood clots: Some studies have suggested that TRT may increase the risk of blood clots, which can be serious or even life-threatening.

Heart problems: TRT may increase the risk of heart attacks, strokes, and other heart problems.

Prostate cancer: There is some evidence that TRT may increase the risk of prostate cancer, although more research is needed to confirm this.

Enlarged prostate: TRT may cause an enlarged prostate, which can lead to urinary symptoms such as difficulty urinating and a frequent need to urinate.

Sleep apnea: TRT may worsen sleep apnea, a condition that causes breathing problems during sleep.

Acne: TRT may cause acne or worsen existing acne.

Breast enlargement: TRT may cause breast enlargement in men, a condition known as gynecomastia.

Reduced sperm production: TRT may reduce sperm production, which can affect fertility.

Mood changes: TRT may cause mood changes, including irritability, aggression, and depression.

Risk of abuse: Testosterone medications are controlled substances, and there is a risk of abuse and dependence with their use.

It's important to discuss the potential risks and benefits of TRT with a healthcare provider before starting treatment

Conclusion

Have you realized that testosterone levels for men peak between the ages of 30 and 35, then begin to decline every year after? What's more, a poor diet can speed up the loss of testosterone production.

Though maintaining a physically active lifestyle, staying hydrated, avoiding smoking and other unhealthy habits, getting enough sleep, and reducing stress are very vital for boosting testosterone levels, one of the key things you can also do to ensure healthy testosterone levels is to eat a healthy diet.

Not all foods are produced equally and when it comes to testosterone, some foods are far better than others. Therefore, it is highly recommended to follow a testosterone diet that is packed with foods that support testosterone production while eliminating estrogenic compounds that are commonly found in foods such as soy.

Let's dive into the best testosterone-boosting recipes and specific foods to begin avoiding and including in your day-to-day diet to optimize your testosterone levels.

The best testosterone-boosting diet is one that will take into consideration these important three factors:

Going Natural: If you want to increase your testosterone through diet, you need to focus on natural and whole food choices while removing processed and unhealthy food choices.

Avoid buying anything that is processed or contains a blend of artificial sweeteners and flavoring.

Knowing Your Calories: You'll never get to where you're going if you don't know the destination. You can take a look at your caloric intake as a road map to guide you to your goals of testosterone production.

Knowing how many calories you need to be eating per day can be essential for ensuring you stay on course and don't overeat, which can lead to obesity and lower testosterone levels.

Avoiding Testosterone-Lowering Foods: Being familiar with the worst foods for testosterone is going to keep you well ahead of the game when it comes to boosting your testosterone.